KT-570-358

THE SHELDON
SHORT GUIDE TO
PHOBIAS
AND **PANIC**

Professor **Kevin Gournay**

sheldon**PRESS**

First published in Great Britain in 2015

Sheldon Press
36 Causton Street
London SW1P 4ST
www.sheldonpress.co.uk

Copyright © Professor Kevin Gournay 2015

All rights reserved. No part of this book may be
reproduced or transmitted in any form or by
any means, electronic or mechanical, including
photocopying, recording, or by any information
storage and retrieval system, without permission in
writing from the publisher.

The author and publisher have made every effort to
ensure that the external website and email addresses
included in this book are correct and up to date at the
time of going to press. The author and publisher are
not responsible for the content, quality or continuing
accessibility of the sites.

British Library Cataloguing-in-Publication Data
A catalogue record for this book is available from the
British Library

ISBN 978-1-84709-368-4
eBook ISBN 978-1-84709-369-1

Typeset by Fakenham Prepress Solutions, Fakenham,
Norfolk NR21 8NN
First printed in Great Britain by Ashford Colour Press
Subsequently digitally reprinted in Great Britain

eBook by Fakenham Prepress Solutions, Fakenham,
Norfolk NR21 8NN

Produced on paper from sustainable forests

Contents

Introduction

'Fear is normal.' I probably use these three words every time I see a new client who comes to me with phobic anxiety or panic. The problem with fear is that, as with many normal phenomena, it can simply get out of hand. Fear can grow into a phobia, so that the presence of a particular object, or being in a particular situation, leads to a level of fear that is unpleasant and overwhelming and makes you want to escape from it at the earliest possible opportunity. Likewise, 'nervousness', which everyone feels on some occasions, can grow to such an extent that we become overwhelmed by a mixture of physical feelings and thoughts of such intensity that we feel like a catastrophe is about to occur – death is imminent, or a loss of control, or madness.

Fear is an essential part of all our lives. If you think about it, people *without* fear would be killed the first time they crossed a road. Ask yourself: 'Is it normal to have some fear and apprehension?' If the choice is walking down a well-lit road or taking a shortcut through a dark underpass late at night, what stops us choosing the riskier route? Fear has a survival function: it protects us from making unwise choices and walking through the dark underpass instead of down the well-lit road. Fear also protects us in a physical sense. The hormone of fear – adrenaline – prepares our body for 'fight or flight' responses to situations.

Phobias and panic may happen when fear gets out of hand, and I deal with these two topics together as they are often inextricably linked. The majority of people I see in outpatient clinics with phobias experience panic attacks, and the pattern of their panic can become as much of a problem as the phobia. In this book I describe a tried and tested self-help programme, which I designed more than 15 years ago.

A key word is **exposure**. To remove phobic fears from your life, you need to face them, and this guide teaches you how to do that.

There is an emphasis on two principles:

1 exposure to phobias and panic needs to be carried out in steps, with you gradually increasing your efforts;
2 exposure should be at a level that you find difficult, but manageable. If you try to push yourself too far, you will suffer setbacks.

I must emphasize that this book will not have all the answers. I do hope, however, that in helping you to help yourself, I can at the very least point you in the right direction.

Part 1

PHOBIAS AND PANIC – THE FACTS

1

Categories of anxiety states

Phobias and panic are **anxiety states**. Anxiety states may be classified into the following groups:

- simple (specific) phobias
- social phobia or social anxiety disorder
- panic and panic disorder
- agoraphobia with and without panic disorder
- generalized anxiety states.

How common are fears and phobias?

As an approximate guide, one in ten of the population has a phobia that would be severe enough to warrant treatment, while approximately 4 per cent have a social phobia, and approximately 5 per cent agoraphobia or agoraphobic-like symptoms. Approximately one in three of the population will experience a panic attack at some time during their lives.

It is clear, therefore, that anxiety states, in various shapes and forms, are very common and nothing to be ashamed of. Being anxious does not mean that you lack courage or are weak. I have had the privilege, in my professional life, of meeting thousands of people with anxiety states. I have nothing but admiration for them as many have exhibited levels of courage that I could never attain, and contribute so much to our community despite their fears.

People with anxiety states often have phobias and panic attacks that need to be treated in their own right. But let's deal first with anxiety states.

Simple (specific) phobias

A phobia may be defined as a marked or persistent fear that is excessive, unreasonable or out of proportion to the danger that the situation or object presents.

In the vast majority of cases, the person is aware that the fear associated with the phobia is excessive and/or unreasonable and may well acknowledge feeling silly or embarrassed about admitting the problem. Virtually every object or situation you can think of can become the object of a phobia.

Simple phobias often start in early childhood, and many of the people I see tell me, 'I have had this fear for as long as I can remember.' Usually there is no clear reason for the phobia to have developed, but sometimes it starts after a specific traumatic event.

The phrase 'simple phobia' does not necessarily imply that all simple phobias are mild. Some simple phobias can cause high levels of fear, extreme stress and tremendous handicaps in terms of daily living.

I should also say that, sometimes, simple phobias are not so simple! They may be quite complex and generate secondary behaviours, such as checking and taking additional precautions. This is particularly the case in phobias such as those of thunder and lightning or vomiting. Further, some simple phobias are really not simple and isolated, but are central to a range of other anxiety-related problems. Also, they may be accompanied by other secondary phobias and a more general state of anxiety and panic.

I cannot possibly mention in this book every phobia that exists – such a list would involve, literally, thousands of objects and situations. Neither will I attempt to provide a name for each phobia. I know, for example, that the specific fear of Friday the 13th is called 'paraskevidekatriaphobia' – this word deriving from the Greek – but you are unlikely to need to know that. In fact, I have never seen anyone who has this particular phobia!

There are a number of common simple phobias, however, some of which include:

- animal phobias
- flying phobia
- heights phobias
- weather phobias
- fear of dentists
- vomiting phobias
- blood, injury and injection phobias
- illness phobias, health anxiety or hypochondriasis

Social phobia or social anxiety disorder

The layperson's perception of social phobia as a form of shyness is, in some senses, correct. It is usually, however, much more than simple shyness.

The American Psychiatric Association's definition of social phobia is that it is a marked and persistent fear of one or more social or performance situations – that is, when a person is exposed to either unfamiliar people or possible scrutiny by others. Such fears are extremely common but, because of their very nature (they principally concern being humiliated or embarrassed), they are greatly under-reported: many people live with their fears for a lifetime.

People may withdraw from social interaction and become loners, and such lifestyles commonly lead to depression.

Many people with agoraphobic fears often also have a marked degree of social phobia, and there is considerable overlap between the two conditions. Indeed, social phobias are often accompanied by other mental health problems.

Panic and panic disorder

Panic is a very difficult concept to define adequately. One of the problems is that everyone is different and what is experienced as a panic attack by one person may simply be a very high level of anxiety for someone else. Perhaps the best working definition of panic is a condition where, in the mind of the person concerned, the anxiety has become uncontrollable. Often, panic and phobias are intertwined.

The American Psychiatric Association, in its *Diagnostic and Statistical Manual of Mental Disorders* (APA, 2013), defined panic as 'a discrete period of intense discomfort in which four or more of the following symptoms developed abruptly and reached a peak within ten minutes'. These symptoms are:

- palpitations, pounding heart or accelerated heart rate
- sweating
- trembling or shaking
- sensations of shortness of breath or smothering
- feelings of choking
- chest pain or discomfort
- nausea or abdominal distress
- feeling dizzy, unsteady, light-headed or faint

- derealization (feelings of unreality) and deperson-
  alization (feelings of being detached from one's self)
- fear of losing control or going crazy
- fear of dying
- numbing or tingling sensations
- chills or hot flushes.

Many people experience not only four of these symptoms but five, seven or even all 13 of them!

Those who experience panic attacks will know that
it is a combination of symptoms such as the above
that makes them feel something dreadful is about to
happen. The feeling of a loss of control is perhaps the
most central preoccupation. Panic attacks can be such
a distressing problem that the lives of many become
dominated, not by the panic itself but by an anticipa-
tion of panic – fear of fear.

Some people experience periods when the panics
come with considerable ferocity and then go away for
no particular reason.

Having panic attacks day in and day out, as is the
case for some, may lead to dejection and physical
exhaustion. Eventually, some people may develop
depression. Another possible consequence of long-
term panic attacks is for people to develop a reliance on
drugs and alcohol. My own research, conducted some
years ago, showed that one in five people who had
panic attacks and agoraphobia were using alcohol at
dangerously high levels. These findings were confirmed
by similar studies carried out in the UK and USA. See
page 49 for more on how to deal with alcohol.

Spontaneous panic

The psychological and chemical processes that underlie
panic attacks are complex. For some people, there may

be a reason for the panic, such as a familiar phobia. However, for other people they just come out of the blue and for no apparent reason.

Many people who have panic attacks are generally very much more physiologically aroused than the general population and seem to produce adrenaline more readily than others. Such individuals may also be sensitive to other physiological factors, which make their arousal system even more vulnerable – for example, being hungry, tired or short of sleep. Some women have panic attacks at certain times in their menstrual cycle, and other attacks may be caused by the hormonal changes of the menopause.

Many people are more prone to having apparently spontaneous panic attacks after indulging in alcohol or drugs the day before.

Agoraphobia with or without panic disorder

Agoraphobia is a condition in which anxiety occurs in specific places or situations where people perceive that escape might be difficult or embarrassing or help might not be readily available. This then leads to their avoiding going out so that they will not have to face the anxiety these places or situations cause, sometimes to such a degree that they become housebound.

Those with agoraphobia have a number of fears, which may include, for example, being away from home, being in a crowd, travelling on public transport, being in a car, standing in a queue, crossing a bridge and so on. Some people only experience panic attacks when confronted with these situations or when they anticipate that they will be. Others, however, may experience recurrent and unexpected panic attacks that seem to occur spontaneously. For example, sometimes they may be sitting at home, quietly watching television or undertaking relatively relaxing activities, when the feelings of panic develop, sometimes gradually, sometimes abruptly.

Agoraphobia usually starts in early adult life, between 20 and 30. Sometimes it starts very suddenly, but it is more usual for the condition to develop in a gradual way, and in some cases to lead to secondary problems, such as poor self-esteem, marital disharmony and depression.

There may be physical symptoms such as palpitations, sweating, a dry mouth, overactivity of the gastrointestinal tract and shaking.

Hyperventilation or overbreathing (see Chapter 7) causes additional symptoms, which can be very frightening. These include pins and needles or tingling, yawning, sighing, feeling light-headed and faint, feeling unable to breathe and, in some cases, muscle spasms. The person may fear he or she is developing a disease such as cancer or multiple sclerosis or is about to collapse and die.

People with agoraphobia may also worry about suddenly losing control, going mad or fainting, running amok, vomiting or becoming incontinent.

Most people know that their fears are irrational. Nevertheless, when the panic attacks come or they are faced with a situation that triggers fear, they are not in control and cannot dispel their fears, so escape from the object or situation causing the phobia seems the only solution.

In addition to specific fears, many people with agoraphobia would describe themselves as being natural worriers and often anticipating, with anxiety, all kinds of life events. Some people with agoraphobia have other substantial mental health problems, including major depressive illnesses, social phobia or obsessive–compulsive disorder (OCD).

As many as one in eight of us may have one or two agoraphobic fears. For example, many people avoid travelling on the underground or other diverse situations because of anxiety.

Generalized anxiety states

Most of us know what it feels like to be extremely anxious or apprehensive about an impending family event or a change at work. Generalized anxiety states (sometimes called **generalized anxiety disorder** or GAD), however, differ from these normal feelings and mean excessive anxiety and worry that interferes with various aspects of people's lives. Such general anxiety commonly accompanies phobias, both simple and complex.

The six central symptoms of generalized anxiety states are:

- restlessness
- being easily fatigued
- difficulty in concentrating or the mind going blank
- irritability
- muscle tension
- sleeplessness.

Generalized anxiety states may cause great impairment of social, occupational and other areas of life. The condition often progresses until people feel downright depressed and dejected.

While some people are, in a sense, born anxious and may have had a lifelong tendency to worry, some generalized anxiety states are triggered by life events. These might be a stressful job, a poor relationship or a major life change. Those affected may well have been previously calm and relaxed.

On occasions, people may experience almost continuous, high levels of anxiety. Such a state may not develop into full-blown panic, however. Likewise, although the anxiety may be severe, people often carry on with their normal routine and do not attempt to avoid any specific situations. Anxiety states such as these are known to go through phases, and sometimes, for no apparent reason, periods of relative calm will be experienced.

People with general anxiety often experience great levels of fatigue and may be diagnosed as having chronic fatigue syndrome. Sadly, many people diagnosed in this way are, in reality, anxious, and this is not managed correctly.

Other related anxiety disorders

I must also mention three other conditions in which phobias and phobic behaviour play important parts, and which often need to be treated in their own right. They are:

- post-traumatic stress disorder
- obsessive–compulsive disorder
- body dysmorphic disorder.

Post-traumatic stress disorder

The medical definition of post-traumatic stress disorder (PTSD) emphasizes that it has resulted from the person being exposed to a traumatic event. PTSD comprises a range of symptoms. Very often people experience recurrent and intrusive recollections, dreams, visual flashbacks, numbing of general responses, or a markedly diminished interest in their usual activities. People very often complain of feeling detached or estranged from others and may see no future for themselves. Other symptoms include sleep disturbance, irritability or anger and finding it hard to concentrate.

The commonest symptom of PTSD is anxiety that is all-pervasive, coupled with avoidance of many varied situations.

Obsessive–compulsive disorder

Obsessive–compulsive disorder (OCD) is one of the anxiety states that often leads to attacks of panic and avoidance behaviour. OCD can take many forms but essentially consists of intrusive, repetitive and distressing thoughts or compulsions, such as washing hands frequently or checking or repeating an activity.

Body dysmorphic disorder

The term body dysmorphic disorder (BDD) was coined by the American Psychiatric Association in 1994 to describe people who have a preoccupation with an imagined defect in their appearance. It is also applied when people have an actual slight physical anomaly and become disproportionately preoccupied with it.

2

Causes and treatments

Adrenaline: the hormone of the fight or flight response

Adrenaline, or epinephrine, is a hormone produced by the two adrenal glands that sit on top of each kidney.

The function of adrenaline is to prepare the body for action and activity in response to dangerous situations. It does this by increasing the supply of oxygen and glucose to the brain and muscles and suppressing other non-essential bodily processes. Thus, adrenaline increases respiration, heart rate and blood pressure. It dilates the pupils so that we can see as much as possible of the environment. It also evokes the primitive response of contracting the muscles at the base of our hairs so that the 'hair stands up on the back of your neck'. In animals this response to danger makes the animal look fiercer, which can help it to scare off predators.

All these physical processes enable the body to function in an optimum state. While many people worry about the various physical changes that follow a release of adrenaline, the body – even in people with serious illnesses – can withstand the effects, no problem. Indeed, adrenaline is injected in emergencies when someone needs to be resuscitated. When the body is under the influence of high levels of adrenaline, the heart muscle is probably working at its optimum efficiency.

People are concerned about the long-term effects of the fight or flight response, also called the stress reaction, but the evidence for anxiety in itself shortening life or causing various illnesses is quite limited. There is even some evidence that anxious people live longer than their relaxed fellows.

What causes anxiety and phobias?

The simple answer is this: nobody can really provide a definitive account of how anxiety and phobias arise.

Brain imaging using MRI (magnetic resonance imaging) scans has shown clearly that certain areas of the brain are implicated in anxiety, and seems to suggest that the brains of those who experience states of anxiety may differ in subtle ways from those of people without anxiety states. There is now a strong probability that a great deal of anxiety may be genetically determined (for example, scientists are fairly certain that there is a substantial genetic component to panic disorder, agoraphobia and obsessive–compulsive disorder).

Research also seems to confirm the long-held view that most people with anxiety are biologically predisposed to reacting in a more marked way physiologically than other people, simply pumping out more adrenaline. This predisposition may combine with other psychological and social factors occurring during childhood and, later in life, a fear or a phobia may develop.

Sometimes, however, when I listen to the history of someone with an anxiety disorder, it becomes clear that it started after a specific trauma. For example, the person may have been involved in an accident or trapped in a lift, or experienced a sudden bereavement or separation.

Finally, social factors, such as poverty, social isolation, unemployment, and social support, are of great importance in the way that anxiety states evolve.

Treatments

The two central approaches to treating phobias and panic, supported by an enormous amount of research evidence, are:

- cognitive behaviour therapy
- medication.

Self-help organizations may also be helpful.

Cognitive behavioural therapy (CBT)

CBT is a process that emphasizes behaviour. Therefore, in overcoming phobias, people change their behaviour by gradually facing something that has previously been avoided. The central treatment technique in CBT for phobias and panic is exposure therapy, which has been shown to be an effective way of tackling the problem.

The IAPT (Improving Access to Psychological Therapies) initiative aims to make CBT more accessible, and there are some effective online programmes. Do ask your GP or practice nurse about this.

Medication

Drug treatments for panic and phobias are as old as history. Indeed, the commonest remedy for all forms of anxiety has been the drug alcohol. It is still very frequently used by those with phobias and panic and can, of course, lead to very serious problems.

Tranquillizers

The most commonly prescribed drug is diazepam (Valium), although several other varieties of benzodiazepines (such as Ativan and Xanax) have also been prescribed in large quantities. The great difficulty with these drugs is that they quickly lead to addiction and their beneficial effect on anxiety wears off after a few dozen doses. In terms of treating panic and phobias, these drugs are not to be recommended.

Over the years, a number of self-help groups, such as Beat the Benzos (<www.benzo.org.uk>), have grown up for people addicted to tranquillizers.

Antidepressants

There are various antidepressants that are marketed for the treatment of anxiety, mainly the selective serotonin reuptake inhibitors (SSRIs), such as Prozac (fluoxetine), Seroxat (paroxetine), Cipramil (citalopram) and Cipralex (escitalopram). There are also drugs related to SSRIs, such as Cymbalta (duloxetine) and Effexor (venlafaxine).

The older tricyclic antidepressants include imipramine and amitriptyline, but have serious long-term side effects, including enormous weight gain and effects on the heart and liver.

Alternative remedies

Many people take natural remedies and homeopathic preparations. While I have no doubt that some people derive benefit from them because of a placebo effect, there is no research evidence for any of these alternative remedies having a place in the treatment of anxiety. My one additional note of caution is that, because natural remedies are unregulated in the UK, you can never be completely sure what it is that you are taking.

Psychotherapy

The theory behind traditional psychotherapeutic treatments is that the symptoms are merely the product of an underlying conflict that often has its roots in childhood. One major difficulty associated with the psychoanalytical explanation of a variety of mental health problems is that they largely ignore any possible biological underpinnings of the problems. They also overlook the many and varied social factors that may be partly responsible for the cause and substantially maintain the difficulty in the longer term.

Self-help organizations

I certainly believe that one of the central principles behind the self-help movement should be the more the merrier! I am the proud president and founding patron of No Panic.

No Panic was set up for those with phobias, panic attacks, obsessive–compulsive disorders, general anxiety disorders and going through tranquillizer withdrawal. It offers a range of services, literature, audio and video cassettes and DVDs. The charity puts people in contact with others and offers a recovery programme delivered via the telephone.

The first port of call for anyone with a health problem should be your GP, who may refer you to a psychiatrist. I would, however, suggest that you first try a self-help programme, such as that outlined in this book. Try and carry it out in a systematic manner for at least three weeks and possibly up to three months.

Part 2

THE SELF-HELP PROGRAMME

The following self-help programme is aimed primarily at those with phobias, but may help with other anxiety problems. The programme consists of the following steps:

1 defining your problem;
2 selecting your targets or goals;
3 deciding on and implementing your plan;
4 dealing with specific phobias;
5 managing panic and general anxiety;
6 evaluating your progress.

Don't try to tackle them all in one go. Take your time. So when, for example, you come to plan your treatment targets, make your list and then sleep on it. Return to your list the following day and ask yourself, 'Have I got that right? Do I need to add something more?' Equally, don't try to achieve the perfect plan. Try things out and, if they don't work out as you wished, take a step back and see how you can improve it.

Then, as I say to all those who come to me to embark on their treatment journeys: don't just think about it, do it!

3

Defining your problem

Defining the precise nature of your problem is the first necessary step on your road to recovery. But it is essential to do this in clear and unambiguous terms.

For example, saying 'simply' that you are agoraphobic or that you have panic attacks does not really describe the problem. It is rather like saying, 'My car is not running properly.' If you took your car to a garage you would provide the mechanic with more information than that – as much as possible, in fact – so that the problem could be diagnosed and sorted out.

You must specify or state what the problem is and how it affects your life. Find the answers to some basic questions, such as:

- What is the nature of your anxiety?
- What physical symptoms do you experience?
- Does your anxiety include certain thoughts, such as 'I'm going to pass out', 'I'm going to collapse' or 'I must escape'?
- Do you use props that make the anxiety better? For example, using a walking stick, carrying a mobile phone or bottle of water may make you feel more secure. (These modifying factors are important because they can be used later in treatment.)
- Do you find some factors make situations worse, such as bright lights in supermarkets, being stuck in

traffic, your menstrual cycle, or times of day such as night or early morning?

For example, someone might define their agoraphobic fear as follows:

- Fear of situations where there is no obvious escape, such as crowded buses, trains, theatres and super-markets. This fear leads to an avoidance of such situations, which in turn restricts my ability to work, shop and socialize.
- The fear comprises thoughts connected with a loss of control (passing out, fainting, vomiting, col-lapsing, becoming incontinent). Although I know that these thoughts are irrational, they can be overwhelming.

It may be helpful to break the problem down in slightly different ways – by making a list of things that are causing you difficulty, for example.

- Try to identify exactly what it is that you are afraid of happening (for example, collapsing, dying, fainting).
- Define the situations that cause the anxiety. When and where does it occur?
- Define how the avoidance of those situations leads to handicap. What effects does it have on you?

Conclusion

Defining your problem is the first step on your road to recovery. Make sure that you do the following:

- Think about all the components that make up your problem.
- Identify those situations that cause you difficulty or that you tend to avoid.
- Define the thoughts that trouble you.
- Identify all those factors that make the problem worse or better.
- Define how the problem upsets and/or interferes with your normal activities.

Once you have done this, use your list as your problem statement, and go on to the next stage, which is to select your treatment targets or goals.

4

Selecting your targets or goals

The very first question you should ask yourself is, 'What would I like to do that I can't do at present because of my problems?'

This is an important question and should be answered honestly. Be selfish: think about what you want; put to one side what you think others expect of you. You need to bear in mind that other people might sometimes want you to do things that you do not necessarily want to do.

Setting your targets should be a two-stage process:

1 decide what goals (targets) you wish to achieve;
2 define each one in detail.

Deciding on your goals or targets

Have another look at your original list of problems to help you see what targets you wish to aim for. For example, if your fear is of underground trains, your target might be to travel to work using the tube. If your problem concerns panic, your target might be to face up to panicky feelings when they occur and use strategies designed to reduce or eliminate your symptoms.

If your problem stops you doing things that you enjoy, such as pursuing your hobbies or interests, you should begin by trying to develop targets that are enjoyable in their own right, but may involve exposure to situations that would normally cause you anxiety. Going to a football match or joining an evening class might be obvious examples.

Defining your targets in detail

As with problem statements, targets need to be specific. This is probably best illustrated by the following example.

Say that one of your targets is to 'Travel by underground train'. This phrase does not tell you very much about the precise behaviour you are aiming for. A more suitable long-term (ultimate) target might be:

> To travel by underground from Arnos Grove Station to Piccadilly Circus, five times a week, in the rush hour. This journey will be undertaken alone, without the aid of the water bottle that I use to deal with the possibility that I might choke. During the journey I will practise observing fellow passengers, rather than distracting myself by listening to my iPod.

Obviously you may wish to develop your target behaviours in a more gradual way. Using the example above, instead your first target might be:

> To travel by underground train from Cockfosters to Southgate station (two stops, no long tunnels) after the rush hour finishes with a friend at least twice a week.

Ideally, each defined problem should have at least three goal (or target) statements attached to it. It does not matter how many targets you set, but it is worth considering how these may be broken down so that you can tackle them in stages. For example, you may choose to set targets to be achieved in the short term (within four weeks), medium term (within three months) and longer term (within six months to a year).

Write your targets down and display them in a place where you will see them frequently.

Conclusion

Drawing up a list of targets is the second step on your road to recovery. Make sure that you do the following:

- make a list of the things that you want to be able to do;
- be very specific about the detail of each target;
- make sure that the target reflects your problem statement;
- think about your targets in the short, medium and long term.

When you have made your list, show it to your spouse, partner or a trusted friend. You should do this so as to check whether or not there are additional targets you might wish to include. This also provides you with an opportunity to enlist support and practical help so that you can achieve your targets.

Keep your list of targets in a place where you will see it frequently.

5

Deciding on and implementing your plan

Exposure to the object or situation causing you anxiety is essential if you are to overcome your fears. This is a central principle of this therapy.

Thus, the central element in your plan must be exposure to that which you fear. Other aspects of anxiety management and control are also important, however, such as paying attention to exercise, diet, time management and alcohol (see Chapter 8).

It is important that your plan is *written down*.

Write down all the aspects of your plan that you can think of and then consider them in the light of any constraints imposed by your normal routine or your life priorities. In my experience, if you are to overcome your phobia, your exposure plan needs to be a top priority in your life. If you cannot decide firmly that the plan is your number one priority, you will probably not succeed in overcoming your fears.

Drawing up your plan

The use of exposure in your imagination and real life

There is ample evidence that using your imagination can be very helpful in the early stages of treatment.

What you need to do is quite simple. Try to imagine

yourself in the situation or facing the object you fear, while at the same time seeing yourself calmly staying there and coping with that situation. This can be a very helpful way to prepare yourself for the real thing.

Most people with phobias will try to push any thoughts about their phobic object from their mind. Try to do the opposite. Try thinking about the situation or object for as long as possible, but at least ten minutes at a time.

Dealing with specific phobias

The same rules of exposure apply to managing specific phobias as to the more complex phobias, such as agoraphobia. Gradual exposure to the feared situation or object is the central approach.

Each type of phobia may call for some additional strategies to deal with problems specific to that phobia. For example, in the case of a vomiting phobia, secondary problems, such as checking behaviours or an obsession with sell-by dates and the state of food in the fridge, would need to be dealt with.

One approach would be to let someone else take responsibility for cooking as he or she might also have a more relaxed attitude to sell-by dates. For someone with such a phobia, giving up control is a real step forward.

Similarly, the person with the phobia may have avoided drinking alcohol. In such a case, I would advise drinking alcohol moderately on a regular basis (see pp. 49–52). Note that this is contrary to my general advice to people with phobias!

To take another example: if someone has a fear of heights, simply trying to conquer taller and taller buildings will probably not be sufficient. The plan should involve a wide range of situations that involve facing this fear – looking out through a window, standing on a balcony, driving across a road bridge, crossing a bridge over water on foot, sitting on a bench at the top of a cliff and so on.

With this fear it is also a good idea to use films and computer programs that feature heights as a means of increasing exposure to them. In general, such strategies are often helpful in preparing the individual concerned for the real thing.

Social phobias present a very wide range of chal-lenges. Not only do social situations have their particular difficulties but also the particular aspects of each person's fear need to be carefully considered. In the example of someone who fears blushing, one might suggest a ban on make-up used to camouflage the blushing skin. It could also be suggested that the person concerned observe others to see them coping with similar problems.

Treatment approaches need to be tailored specifi-cally to both the phobia in question and the individual circumstances.

How often should I expose myself to the object or situation causing the phobia, and for how long?

Research shows very clearly that long sessions of exposure are much more effective than short ones. That is because, put simply, you need to allow yourself time to calm down.

You will feel you are beginning to calm down after a few minutes, but to have a lasting effect on reducing your anxiety often takes much longer. So the longer you can stay in the situation the better, because your body can only keep up high levels of adrenaline output for relatively brief periods. In addition, the longer your exposure continues, the more you will realize that what you fear will not happen.

Ideally, then, exposure sessions should last two hours. Although this may sound like a tall order, there is a great deal of evidence to show that this amount of time is much more effective than shorter periods of 30 minutes or so. Regular practice is important too.

The simple rule of thumb is that, if at all possible, you should face your fears on a daily basis. My experience is that doing so as much as you possibly can will always be more helpful than being conservative. I believe that there is very little risk from frequent sessions and that, although many people anticipate that they may 'overdo it', that is unlikely.

How gradual should my exposure be?

Some people can progress very quickly to facing their most feared object or situation; others may take a little longer. People are different! Some folk can very quickly graduate to doing the worst thing that they can imagine (for example, travelling on a crowded underground train in the rush hour), while others need to approach their fears very gradually.

Research does not really reveal any conclusive evidence either way. A simple rule of thumb is to do what is difficult, but just about manageable.

Do I need to experience anxiety during exposure sessions?

Although most people dread exposure treatment and anticipate that they will have very high levels of anxiety, the amount they experience when they confront their feared situation or object is very variable. Indeed, a significant minority of people experience very little anxiety when they eventually face up to a situation that they may have avoided for many years.

The simple answer is that, in terms of overcoming your phobia, it does not seem to matter how much anxiety you experience during an exposure session, provided you continue to have exposure sessions as often and for as long as you can.

Going it alone versus working with others

There is research to show that for some individuals group treatment sessions can be very effective in helping to overcome phobias and panic. Facing your fears with others often provides additional confidence, motivation and reinforcement. Many of the treatment programmes I have run in hospital outpatient settings have involved group approaches. The camaraderie and friendships that develop are very positive; so is support from a self-help organization such as No Panic. Group treatment is not for everybody, though, and some people simply wish to do it on their own.

Remember also that although you should accept as much practical help as possible from others, your ultimate goal is to be able to face your phobic situations or objects alone. Having someone with you should be seen as an intermediate step on the way. Excessive dependence on others may eventually be detrimental.

Do I need a professional therapist?

The straightforward answer to this question is generally 'no'. Provided that you can follow the central principle of facing your fears, and those around you are supportive, following a plan of increasing exposure may be as good as receiving help from a professional therapist. Professional therapists can provide an objective assessment of your problem, however, and encouragement to face the situation or object.

Having a cotherapist (a partner to work with you)

Most people with phobias and panic receive considerable help from others, but unless it is carefully thought through, such help can at times be counterproductive. For example, the spouse or partner of someone with agoraphobia may take on a number of the responsibilities that that person would normally undertake for himself or herself. In the end, such a shift in responsibilities may be detrimental and counterproductive, promoting an increased dependency on others. The partner may also get drawn into giving endless and meaningless reassurance.

It is not always easy to break old habits, so the treatment plan may have to involve the cotherapist gradually changing his or her behaviour as well. The role of your cotherapist is to provide encouragement and assistance, help you face up to your feared and avoided situations or objects and, at the same time, provide ongoing support and encouragement. This, like many other things, is easier said than done. There will, of course, be pitfalls. If, however, you and your cotherapist review progress objectively, perhaps using the diaries described in the next chapter, many of these pitfalls may be avoided.

6

Keeping a diary

There are numerous ways in which you can keep a diary, but three examples are provided below.

The first is a general diary (see Table 1), wherein day-to-day activities and ratings as to the level of your anxiety and mood are noted. Recording such information over a period of time will help you to see the relationships between what you do and how you feel. The 'Comments' section on the far right can be used to summarize your overall view of the day.

Table 1 Example of a general diary

Date	Main events of the day	High/low anxiety points*	Mood ratings**	Comments

Notes
* Score anxiety on a scale from 0 to 8, where 0 = no anxiety and 8 = worst anxiety possible.
**Score depression on a scale from 0 to 8, where 0 = no problems and 8 = worst depression possible.

The second type of diary – an exposure diary – is specific to exposure tasks and is used to record the length of your sessions and your anxiety ratings (see Table 2).

You should record your anxiety ratings before, during and after a session. It is also important to note whether or not a cotherapist has been present, and then to plan your next task.

This simple format can be modified and extra columns added as required.

Table 2 Example of an exposure diary

Date	Exposure situation	Length of session	Anxiety ratings*	Cotherapist present?	Next task planned

Note
* Score anxiety on a scale from 0 to 8, where 0 = no anxiety and 8 = worst possible anxiety.

The thoughts diary (see Table 3) can be particularly valuable for those who experience panic attacks, as it helps you to identify various patterns of negative and catastrophic thoughts.

This is an important process that acts as a first step in managing the thoughts associated with panic attacks. Various strategies that you can adopt are described in the next chapter.

Table 3 Example of a thoughts diary

Date	Situation	Triggers	Thoughts	Consequences

Overall, diaries of how you feel, what you do and how successful you are provide perhaps the best way to evaluate your progress. You should keep your original list of problems and targets and use the diaries as a way of determining how close you are to achieving the targets you have set for yourself.

It may well be that, after a while, your targets need to be revised and, indeed, it may become clear as you go on that your view of your problem changes. In this case, you will need to revise your original definition (see Chapter 3). This often happens when you have avoided something for a long time, and it is not until you begin to face it that you start to see things in a different light.

7

Managing panic and general anxiety

Managing panic

Panic management essentially comprises three central approaches. The first, and perhaps the most important, is

1 to maintain exposure. That means you should prevent yourself from 'escaping' from the situation.

Then we have:

2 dealing with hyperventilation;
3 dealing with catastrophic thoughts.

Hyperventilation

As we have seen, when we become anxious, our body's reaction is to prepare for 'fight or flight'. One element of this reaction is that we breathe more rapidly to provide the body with the additional oxygen it requires. In a state of anxiety and panic, however, the increase in our breathing rate is not required to help us to fight or flee from our foe! We are, in effect, breathing in excess of what our body actually needs.

Over time such hyperventilation (sometimes also called **overbreathing**) will lead to an imbalance in body chemistry. That is because there will be a reduction in carbon dioxide levels, leading to sensations such as pins and needles, feeling light-headed, yawning or sighing and, in extreme cases, muscle spasms. Hyperventilating for extended periods of time also causes fatigue and sleepiness.

For those who have panic attacks, the symptoms produced by hyperventilation are frightening in themselves and, taken with other symptoms of anxiety, such as a rapid heart rate, they may feel that they are just about to have a stroke or a heart attack. As a result, the body produces more adrenaline, which in turn makes matters worse by feeding into a downward spiral of anxiety.

There is considerable evidence to show that teaching people to breathe more appropriately can be very effective in helping to reduce hyperventilation. The difficulty for some people is that panic develops so abruptly they do not realize that they are doing it.

Dealing with hyperventilation

Hyperventilation usually leads to breathing being shallow, restricted to the upper part of the chest, and rapid.

Simple breathing exercises, consisting of taking slow, but not too deep, breaths, can be extremely helpful. Ensuring that your breathing comes from the diaphragm, rather than from the top of your chest, is very important. You can check that you are achieving this by placing your hand on your abdomen, slightly below your ribcage. Your tummy should move in and out to ensure that as much of the chest as possible is used.

Generally speaking, people who hyperventilate can reverse the pattern of overbreathing by practising the slow diaphragmatic breathing described above once

What to do in the case of acute panic

Hyperventilation can sometimes lead to an acute panic attack. If possible, try to find somewhere quiet to either sit or lie down and endeavour to take slow breaths, breathing slowly from the diaphragm. It is helpful to loosen your clothing and relax your posture. Although this can be very difficult, try to concentrate on relaxing your muscles and, at the same time, remember that panic can do no real harm.

One very rapid and effective way to deal with the hyperventilation associated with panic is the old tried and tested method of rebreathing exhaled air. Exhaled air contains more carbon dioxide than the air around us, so rebreathing it replenishes the carbon dioxide in your body, thus reversing the chemical changes that follow from hyperventilation, as described above.

You can rebreathe exhaled air by breathing in and out of a paper bag, the top gathered in one hand and placed over your mouth. If this is not possible, a simple alternative is to cup your hands over your nose and mouth and rebreathe your exhaled air in that way. Doing this for two or three minutes is generally enough to restore the correct chemical balance in the body.

If you are with someone who is hyperventilating, one of the key principles is to remain calm yourself. It is important to remember that hyperventilation, though it can look quite dramatic, is usually self-limiting and very rarely has any serious medical consequences. Very occasionally it can lead to muscular spasm, but this in itself is also harmless and self-limiting. It is the body's way of stopping overbreathing until the chemical balance is restored. Stay with the person and try to ensure that he or she remains still. Try to help the person relax and emphasize the need to breathe slowly and from the diaphragm. Use the paper-bag or cupped-hands techniques described above so that the person can rebreathe his or her exhaled air.

or twice a day, combining this, if possible, with a period of physical relaxation. They should also try to undertake physical exercise (such as running, cycling, swimming, walking) daily.

Dealing with catastrophic thoughts

If you keep a record of your panic attacks, perhaps using a diary (see p. 35), you will find that the thoughts accompanying such attacks will be much the same each time. For most people, the central theme tends to be the fear of some sort of loss of control. For example, you may fear that you will faint, have a stroke or a heart attack, vomit, go mad or die.

One of the most important ways to deal with such catastrophic thoughts is to examine the evidence. For example, you may have panicked on numerous occasions but when did this lead to anything other than anxiety about what could happen? Did you have a heart attack? Did you faint?

Here is a range of strategies that might assist in keeping your thinking balanced.

- Write down a list of pros and cons – that is, points for and against the catastrophic outcome occurring. Then you can make up some small cards to carry in your wallet or purse to read if you feel panicky.
- Record some rational, coping statements on a media player and listen to them in, for example, a crowded train carriage where the panic attacks occur.
- Deliberately bring the thoughts on. It may sound very perverse, but give it a try – it often works. Psychologists and psychiatrists call this method paradoxical intention. Research by anxiety disorder experts has shown that facing these thoughts gives people a feeling that they are in control, rather than

the thoughts controlling them, and so they feel much more able to tackle such patterns of thoughts than they did previously.

Panic is harmless

Remember that panic is harmless and self-limiting, and other people are usually completely unaware that anything is happening. Also, in the longer term, escaping will only make the panic worse. Try and stay in the situation, however hard that seems, breathe slowly and repeat to yourself that nothing will happen. Recall your past experiences – although you may have thought that a heart attack or stroke was imminent, it has never happened. Remind yourself, too, that the body can only pump out adrenaline for brief periods of time, and your symptoms are likely to be due to the high levels of adrenaline rather than anything more sinister.

8

Lifestyle measures for managing general anxiety

For those with phobias and panic, there are five important general areas of lifestyle to consider:

- exercise
- relaxation
- alcohol
- diet
- time management.

Exercise

There is plentiful evidence to suggest that regular and sensible exercise reduces the risk of a very wide range of diseases, and people who exercise regularly report a reduction in their levels of anxiety, tension and depression. Indeed, the National Institute for Health and Care Excellence (NICE) recommends regular aerobic exercise as a first-line treatment for mild to moderate depression.

All forms of exercise, from gardening or playing golf to walking, are to be encouraged. Research suggests very strongly that, for exercise to be effective in making us less susceptible to physical illnesses and to improve our mood and reduce tension, it needs to be at a reasonable level of intensity and repeated at least five times each week.

What is reasonable intensity?

The answer is exercise that maintains 70 to 80 per cent of your maximum heart rate.

How do I calculate my maximum heart rate?

The answer is simple. Maximum heart rate is calculated as 220 minus your age. Therefore, for a 20-year-old, the maximum heart rate is 200 and 70 to 80 per cent of his or her maximum heart rate is therefore 140 to 160 beats per minute.

One of the simplest ways to determine whether or not you are exercising strenuously enough is the talking test. If you are exercising at around 70 to 75 per cent of your maximum heart rate, you should be able to hold a con-versation, but somewhat out of breath and perspiring.

Before embarking on any exercise, and particularly if you have any health problems, are over 40 and have not exercised for a number of years, consult your GP.

How to get started

Do not go straight into a programme of five-times-a-week exercise that gets your heart beating at 70 to 75 per cent of its maximum. Build up to this gradually. You might start by simply walking and jogging for 20 minutes at a time, three times a week, gradually building up your stamina, increasing your exercise by 10 per cent per week.

To achieve this, you need to engage in activities such as running, rowing, cycling, swimming or using a cross-trainer at a gym. Ideally you should mix these different activities so that you exercise different parts of your body. Swimming is great for increasing supple-ness and use of the cross-trainer will exercise your arms and legs. Note that you will not attain the required improvement to your heart rate by going for a gentle stroll in the country, playing a leisurely game of golf or pushing a shopping trolley around the supermarket.

Exercising on your own is difficult, particularly in the dark winter months. Exercising with a friend will keep you motivated. Leisure centres and gyms often have excellent facilities and employ qualified fitness instructors who will usually be able to offer you assistance with an exercise plan. There is some cost involved, but this is a worthwhile investment in your health. You could try group classes, too, such as spinning, which uses static cycles, or aerobics classes.

The Exercise on Prescription Programme

The majority of those with anxiety and panic will probably be eligible for the Exercise on Prescription Programme. This scheme generally operates for people over 15 who have some of the risk factors associated with coronary heart disease.

The programme, which is funded by the government, can also be offered to people to improve mobility, help with the control of diabetes and, most relevant to readers of this book, assist with the treatment of depression.

To find out if you qualify for this programme, simply ask your GP to refer you.

I am too busy to exercise

I am sure that every health professional who has advocated exercise as a remedy for anything at all has heard this plaintive cry. My simple response to this is that the week consists of 168 hours and exercising five times a week for 30 minutes, with some additional time for travelling there and back, getting changed and showering afterwards, will take something in the order of seven to eight hours. That is two and a half hours of exercise and four and a half hours or so of travel and preparation. That still leaves 160 hours in the week.

My simple view is that if you can't give up something in the order of 5 per cent of your overall time to one of the most valuable life activities, then there is surely something wrong with your life. Work out how many hours you spend in front of the TV, channel hopping, and how long you spend – either at work or at home – staring into space or surfing the Internet.

Relaxation

Although relaxation is not used directly as a treatment for either phobias or panic attacks, it can often be helpful in reducing the general level of physical arousal and body tension. The instructions that follow give you an introduction if you want to have a try. Otherwise, there are various relaxation exercises available on CDs or in other forms.

Relaxation training

Relaxation training is a helpful way to reduce the consequences of anxiety and panic.

While there are many ways to achieve relaxation, most focus on a systematic tensing and relaxing of the muscles in the body.

First of all, identify a time in the day when you have 30 minutes to devote to this task. Find a quiet room, unplug or turn off the phone and wear loose, comfortable clothing. The exercise can be carried out in a comfortable chair or lying down.

Get in position and begin with your right hand. Clench your fist so that your knuckles are white. Hold for five seconds then release immediately.

Pause, wait ten seconds, then repeat.

Tense your right forearm, closing your fist and tensing the muscles of your forearm – not too hard. Hold for five seconds then release immediately.

Pause, wait ten seconds, then repeat.

Tense your right biceps, clenching your fist and bending your arm so it forms a 90-degree angle. Concentrate on making your biceps bulge as much as possible. Hold for five seconds then release immediately.

Pause, wait ten seconds, then repeat.

Repeat these actions with the left hand, forearm and biceps, remembering to do each exercise twice, hold for five seconds then release immediately.

Next, move to your head and neck. Tense your eye muscles. Screw up your eyes and keep them shut tight. Hold for five seconds then release immediately.

Pause, wait ten seconds, then repeat.

Tense your mouth by clenching your jaws together and concentrate on pressing your lips together as firmly as possible. At the same time you will notice that you tense your eyes. Hold for five seconds then release immediately.

Pause, wait ten seconds, then repeat.

Now concentrate on tensing your neck. Push your chin down a little towards your chest, but do not touch your chest. Hold for five seconds then release immediately.

Pause, wait ten seconds, then repeat.

Next, move to your shoulders and back, pushing your shoulders up slightly and tensing your neck. Feel the muscles tighten across your shoulders. Hold for five seconds then release immediately.

Pause, wait ten seconds, then repeat.

Tense your shoulders and arms by pushing your arms down, holding your neck rigid. Concentrate on tensing across your shoulders. Hold for five seconds then release immediately.

Pause, wait ten seconds, then repeat.

Tense the muscles in your back by pushing your elbows into your sides, pulling your shoulders down, holding your neck tight and pushing your head down towards your chest. All the time concentrate on tensing the muscles across your back. Hold for five seconds then release immediately.

Pause, wait ten seconds, then repeat.

Now move to your chest and abdomen. Tense the muscles of your chest by pushing your shoulders back, pushing your elbows down into your waist and tilting your head back slightly. Concentrate on holding your chest in a barrel-like rigid way. Hold for five seconds then release immediately.

Pause, wait ten seconds, then repeat.

Tense the muscles of your stomach from the back and pull in towards your navel. Hold for five seconds then release immediately.

Pause, wait ten seconds, then repeat.

Next, move to your lower body and legs. Tense your thighs and buttocks by pushing your buttocks down and concentrate on tensing your thighs and buttocks together. Hold for five seconds then release immediately.

Pause, wait ten seconds, then repeat.

Tense your right calf by pulling your toes up towards you, keeping your leg straight at the knee. Pull your toes back until you can feel the pull all the way up your calf muscles. Hold for five seconds then release immediately.

Pause, wait ten seconds, then repeat.

Tense your right foot by curling over your toes,

trying to make your toes clench like a fist. Hold for five seconds then release immediately.

Pause, wait ten seconds, then repeat.

Repeat this sequence for your left calf and foot.

When you come to this point, begin to tense your whole body, starting with your hands, working up through your arms, then head, neck, shoulders, back, chest, stomach, buttocks, thighs, calves and feet. Take ten seconds to gradually tense the whole body. Hold for five seconds then relax.

As you relax, breathe out as much as you can, slowly. Keep your eyes closed and say 'calm' to yourself.

Repeat this sequence five times, remembering to leave ten seconds between each.

Slow your breathing

Next, concentrate on slowing down your breathing. Try to fill all your chest and, as you breathe out, say the word 'calm' to yourself. Let your breathing settle into a natural rhythm and then try to fix your mind on a quiet and relaxing scene. Imagine yourself lying on a beach or in a meadow. Imagine a warm atmosphere around you. Try to imagine the smells of this environment. Keep your mind as fixed on this place as possible and let yourself drift as much as you can. Don't worry if you fall asleep, but perhaps it may be worth setting your alarm clock first!

Alcohol

Alcohol is the most widely used drug in our society. For many, the effects are very pleasant and, indeed, beneficial.

It is often used as an instant solution to anxiety but, if used to excess, alcohol will make your anxiety much worse and lead to a terrible vicious circle. Research has shown that up to 20 per cent of people with agoraphobia may be using alcohol at dangerously high levels. Some surveys have shown that as many as one in three people admitted to alcohol treatment facilities also have a problem with phobias or panic.

Answer the following questions about your drinking habits.

- Do you drink every day?
- Has your tolerance of alcohol changed? Are you drinking more than before to get the same effect?
- Has your capacity for alcohol increased or decreased?
- Do you feel guilty because of your drinking?
- Do you have memory gaps?
- Do friends comment on the amount you drink?
- Do you sometimes feel shaky after a heavy drinking session?
- Do you exceed the safe drinking limit?

There is some controversy over exactly how much is a safe drinking limit. A rough guide, though, and according to current government advice, is that it is safe to drink between 20 and 30 units a week for a man and 15 to 20 units for a woman. A unit is half a pint of beer, a pub measure of spirits or a small (125 ml) glass of 9 per cent strength wine. A very useful website is <www.at-bristol.org.uk/Alcoholandyou/Facts/units.html>.

If you answered 'yes' to any of the above questions, you really need to think about modifying your drinking. One of the great difficulties with answering the questions honestly is that those who have, or who may be developing, an alcohol problem often rationalize their circumstances. They may say, 'I wouldn't drink as much if my boss was nicer to me', 'Anyone would drink if they had my pressures', or 'I have to drink to help me cope with my problem or my anxiety/depression'.

There are some important principles you can follow that will help to ensure your drinking remains enjoyable and without problematic consequences. They are as follows:

- Give yourself an allowance, not exceeding 20 units per week if you are a man, 15 units if you are a woman.
- Always aim to have at least two to three alcohol-free days in any one week and, once or twice a year, give up alcohol for a week or two. Lent is a good time for some.
- Space your drinks. Try to ensure that you never consume more than one unit per half an hour. If you are at a wedding or party that goes on for several hours, do this by drinking non-alcoholic drinks in between or dilute your wine with mineral water or your beer with lemonade.
- Never drink alone.
- Unless it is a social event that is out of the ordinary, never drink during the day.
- Do not drink during working hours.

Try to apply these principles seriously. Use a diary to record your drinking and do this as honestly and accurately as you can. If after three months you are still answering 'yes' to the questions above, you should certainly seek medical advice or go to one of the local alcohol advisory centres. In more severe cases, it may be that you need the help of Alcoholics Anonymous. You can either visit its website – at <www.alcoholics-anonymous.org.uk> – or the address of your local AA group can be found at your GP's surgery, library or in the telephone book.

Diet

It is not uncommon for those who have panic attacks to eat badly, but a hurried eating pattern and an unbalanced diet may actually make your problem worse.

For someone who is already under stress, problems can be compounded by high quantities of fat or refined sugar as they may lead to rapid variations in blood sugar levels. Indeed, it has been known for many years that some people who experience panic attacks may be prone to dips in blood sugar levels (hypoglycaemia), which may in turn lead to further anxiety.

Some people with anxiety states also hurry their meals, thus causing physical symptoms and long-term digestive problems. It is, therefore, worth considering the advice given in this list.

- Remember to take plenty of time to enjoy your meals – try not to rush them. Allow yourself at least 30 minutes to eat a meal.
- Reduce the speed at which you eat. Put your knife and fork down between mouthfuls, concentrating instead on chewing and enjoying the taste.
- Eat plenty of carbohydrates – pasta, bread, rice and potatoes.
- Ensure that your diet contains sufficient fibre – this will help you to feel satisfied for longer. Eat unrefined carbohydrates, such as wholemeal or granary bread, eat potatoes with their skins left on, eat beans and pulses and have dried and fresh fruits as snacks.
- Avoid refined foods, such as sugar, white bread and fast foods.

- Eat five portions of fresh fruit and vegetables every day.
- Reduce your fat intake – grill foods rather than fry them, use skimmed rather than full-fat milk and substitute low-fat cheeses for full-fat varieties or else eat full-fat cheeses only once or twice a week.
- Try to eat three or four meals a day, making sure that you start with a good breakfast – fruit and cereal are good!
- Avoid snacks but, if you must, eat fruit and vegetables (dried, frozen or fresh).
- Eat with a companion if you can.
- Don't eat your last meal too late at night, and try, if possible, to take a gentle walk after you have eaten.

Omega 3

Over the past 20 years, research into the metabolism of the brain has demonstrated that essential fatty acids called Omega 3 seem to be associated with better mental health.

These fatty acids are found in fish, and it has been noted that in communities that consume fish in high quantities there is a lower overall incidence of mental illness.

The benefits of Omega 3 to cardiac health have been known about for many years. An increasing amount of evidence now demonstrates that it also seems to benefit people who suffer from depression and schizophrenia.

Ethyl EPA, a concentrated form of Omega 3, is available as an over-the-counter supplement called Veg EPA, which is completely free of any of the toxins that contaminate ordinary fish oils.

The evidence concerning the link between EPA and good mental health is very clear.

Time management

Many people with anxiety states feel great pressure and urgency and may have high levels of irritability and anger. They often seem to be attempting to do more than is realistic and are forever trying to put a proverbial quart into a pint pot. This pattern obviously leads to very high levels of stress.

Here are several principles that you should follow to ensure that you manage your time effectively.

- Set yourself reasonable and attainable goals. Set ones for the short, medium and long term. Accept, however, that some of your goals may not be attained.
- Ensure that your goals cover all areas of your life, not just work or household duties. Remember to include your hobbies and personal interests.
- Set daily and weekly priorities. Try to list all the things that you want to do in a week and then decide which are the most important.
- Remember that we can never achieve all that we want to achieve. Be reasonable and realistic about the priorities you set for yourself.
- Set aside a reasonable amount of time for each activity and allow for unexpected interruptions. Try to plan each day so that you work on your priorities, but remember that life often throws up unexpected interruptions. Some flexibility is, therefore, required.

Time management is based on such simple common-sense principles. The first major element is recognizing that you may put too much pressure on yourself. Most people with time management problems are pressured by themselves rather than others. Taking the pressure off yourself will help you to feel more relaxed so that, in the long run, your susceptibility to anxiety will be decreased.

9

Evaluating your progress

The most reliable way to evaluate your progress is to use your problem and target definitions, sit down with a friend, partner or spouse (or cotherapist) and decide how much progress you have made towards your targets.

Furthermore, a simple recording of your day-to-day behaviour in a diary is the final arbiter of success.

The examples of diaries in Chapter 6 showed an anxiety scale, ranging from 0 to 8, to help you record the strength of your feelings of anxiety. Changes in these scores over time also enable you to see how you have progressed. You should not expect your anxiety ratings to drop dramatically when you start a self-help programme, but, if you are facing the phobic situation regularly, they should gradually decrease.

If after, say, ten exposures there is no real reduction in your anxiety, you need to think again about whether or not these sessions are being properly carried out. One common reason for failing to make progress is that your sessions are not long enough. Or, change the focus of your exposure, perhaps concentrating for a while on those parts of your plan that are more successful and returning to the more difficult part(s) when you have had more success.

If you haven't been keeping a diary, take another look at Chapter 3, work through the points on defining your problem and deciding what your targets are, then, using the examples provided, draw up a diary that is suitable for you.

Conclusion

- Look at your original targets.
- Take each in turn and assess what progress you have made.
- Don't worry too much if you are doing better in some areas than others.
- If there is a particular sticking point, leave it alone for a while and return to it later.
- Expect some improvement in your anxiety ratings, but assume that progress may be slow and there will be occasions when you experience setbacks.

The central message is that you must persist with your exposure sessions and try to keep to your plan. Don't be afraid to reconsider your list of problems and targets and adjust your plan if need be: then take the appropriate action.

Conclusion:
You really can do it!

Fears and phobias are, in my opinion, an integral part of the human condition. In the UK, the number of people who have fears and phobias, at a level that causes upset to everyday life, is not thousands or hundreds of thousands but millions. It is clear that it will never be possible to provide professional help for all these people, even if we had the most utopian of healthcare systems.

Having said that, it is also clear to me, after 30-plus years working in the field, that many people have anxiety problems but, for whatever reason, do not want to be treated by a professional. In my opinion, for these people and others, self-help is a greatly under-rated method for dealing with fears and phobias. An increasing amount of research evidence has concluded that, for some people, self-help is as effective or even more effective than professional interventions delivered by highly trained individuals.

I appreciate that not all of the suggestions given in this book will suit all those with fears and phobias. If that is the case for you, I would suggest you identify those parts of the book you have found to be helpful and concentrate on those sections. One thing it is crucial to remember, though, is that exposure to what you fear is a non-negotiable precondition for overcoming your fears and phobias, and should be central to whatever you do. I appreciate that facing your fears and phobias will usually involve a measure of anxiety and distress, but the old maxim 'No pain, no gain' is true for the vast majority of people who embark on a programme of either self-help or professional treatment.

One of the most important lessons I have learned is that each person with a fear or a phobia is different from the next. There is no formula for any problem; everyone is different. There is certainly no magic formula for recovery either. One of the most important things in my professional life, however, has been the satisfaction that I have derived from seeing people overcome sometimes apparently insurmountable levels of fear and anxiety. Whatever your fears or phobias may be, you must know one simple truth: there is every reason to hope that you, too, will overcome them.